Daily Keto Recipes

Simple And Healthy Recipes For Busy People On A Keto Diet

Elena Harrison

Table of Contents

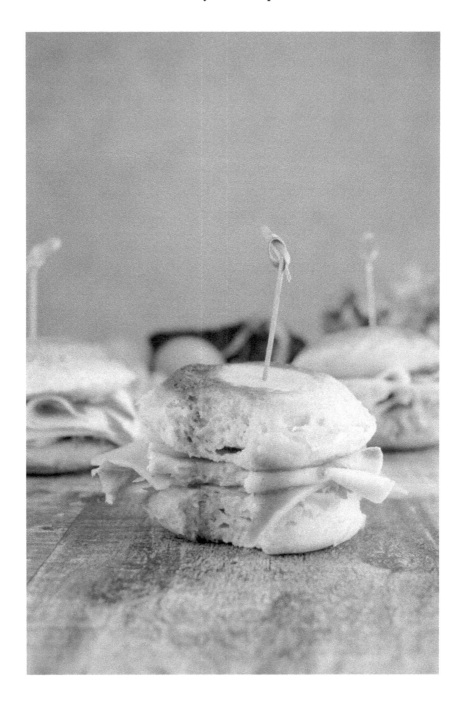

INTRODUCTION

The ketogenic diet has been highly praised and praised for the benefits of weight loss. This high-fat, low-carb diet has been shown to be extremely healthy overall. It really makes your body burn fat, like a talking machine. Public figures appreciate it too. But the question is, how does ketosis enhance weight loss? The following is a detailed picture of the ketosis and weight loss process.

Some people consider ketosis to be abnormal. Although it has been approved by many nutritionists and doctors. many people still disapprove of it. The misconceptions are due to the myths that have spread around the ketogenic diet.

Once your body is out of glucose, it automatically depends on stored fat. It is also important to understand that carbohydrates produce glucose and once you start a low carbohydrate diet, you will also be able to lower your glucose levels. Then your body will produce fuel through fat, instead of carbohydrates, that is, glucose.

The process of accumulating fat through fat is known as ketosis, and once your body enters this state, it becomes extremely effective at burning unwanted fat. Also, since glucose levels are low during the ketogenic diet, your body achieves many other health benefits.

A ketogenic diet is not only beneficial for weight loss, but it also helps improve your overall health in a positive way. Unlike all other diet plans, which focus on reducing calorie intake, ketogenic focuses on putting your body in a natural metabolic state, that is, ketosis. The only factor that makes this diet questionable is that this nature of metabolism is not very well thought out. By getting tattoos on your body regularly, your body will quickly burn stored fat, leading to great weight loss.

Now the question arises. How does ketosis affect the human body?

However, this phase does not last more than 2-3 days. This is the time it takes for the human body to enter the ketosis phase. Once you get in, you won't have any side effects.

You should also start gradually reducing your calorie and carbohydrate intake. The most common mistake dietitians make is that they tend to start eliminating everything from their diet at the same time. This is where the problem arises. The human body will react extremely negatively when you limit everything at once. You must start gradually. Read this guide to learn more about how to approach the ketogenic diet after 50.

Most fats are good and essential for our health so there are essential fatty acids and essential amino acids (proteins). Fat is the most efficient form of energy, and each gram contains about 9 calories. This more than doubles the amount of carbohydrates and protein (both have 4 calories per gram).

When you eat a lot of fat and protein and significantly reduce carbohydrates, your body adjusts and converts the fat and protein, as well as the fat that it has stored, into ketones or ketones, for energy. This metabolic process is called ketosis. This is where the ketogen in the ketogenic diet comes from.

BREAKFAST

1. Almond Pancakes

Preparation Time: 5 minutes

Cooking Time: 15 minutes

Servings: 2

Ingredients:

- ½ cup almond flour
- 1 egg
- 2 ½ tablespoons unsweetened almond milk
- 2 tablespoons coconut oil, divided (1 tablespoon for batter, 1 tablespoon for frying)
- 1 tablespoon erythritol (optional; use if you want sweet taste)
- Pinch salt (if using sweetener)
- ½ teaspoon baking powder
- ½ teaspoon pure vanilla extract (optional)

Directions:

1. In a bowl, put and mix all the ingredients except 1 tablespoon of coconut oil with a whisk until smooth.
2. Place an oiled pan over medium-low heat. Pour heaping tablespoons of batter onto the pan and form pancakes. Cover and fry about 1-2 minutes, then flip pancakes when bubbles start to form and cook another 1-2 minutes.

3. Transfer pancakes to the plate and repeat the cooking process until the batter is used up.
4. Serve whipped cream or sour cream and berries (do not forget about carbs in berries and cream).

Nutrition: Calories: 325 Total Carbs: 7g Fiber: 4g Net Carbs: 3g Fat: 30g Protein: 9g

2. Cottage Cheese Pancakes

Preparation Time: 5 minutes

Cooking Time: 15 minutes

Servings: 2

Ingredients:

- cheese
- 2 eggs
- ½ tablespoon psyllium husk powder
- 4 ounces heavy whipping cream
- 1 ounce coconut oil (or butter) for frying

Directions:

1. Mix cottage cheese, eggs and psyllium husk powder in a bowl, until well combined. Set the mixture aside for 5-7 minutes to thicken.
2. Place an oiled pan over medium-low heat. Pour 2-inch circles of batter onto the pan and try to make small–sized pancakes. It's easier to flip smaller pancakes. Fry pancakes for 2-4 minutes on both sides until golden brown.
3. In another bowl, whip heavy cream to soft peaks.
4. Serve the cottage cheese pancakes with whipped cream and enjoy!

Nutrition: Calories: 473 Total Carbs: 7g Fiber: 2g Net Carbs: 5g Fat: 43g Protein: 16g

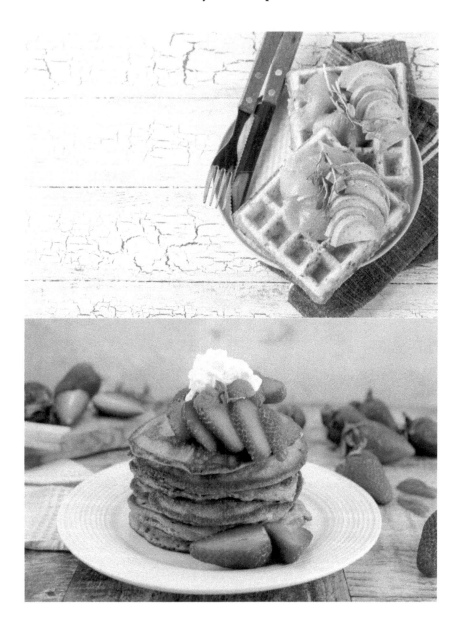

KETO BREAD

3. Low-Carb Blueberry English muffin Bread Loaf

Preparation Time: 4 minutes

Cooking Time: 14 min

Serving: 5

Ingredients:

- 1/2 cup almond spread or cashew or nutty spread
- 1/4 cup spread ghee or coconut oil
- 1/2 cup almond flour
- 1/2 tsp. salt
- 2 tsp. preparing powder
- 1/2 cup almond milk unsweetened
- 5 eggs beaten
- 1/2 cup blueberries

Directions:

1. Preheat stove to 350 degrees F.
2. In a microwavable bowl dissolve nut margarine and spread together for 30 seconds, mix until joined well.
3. In a huge bowl, whisk almond flour, salt, and heating powder together. Empty the nut spread blend into the huge bowl and mix to consolidate.

4. Whisk the almond milk and eggs together at that point fill the bowl and mix well.
5. Drop-in new blueberries or break separated solidified blueberries and tenderly mix into the hitter.
6. Line a portion dish with material paper and daintily oil the material paper also.
7. Pour the hitter into the portion dish and prepare 45 minutes or until a toothpick in focus confesses all.
8. Cool for around 30 minutes at that point expel from container.
9. Slice and toast each cut before serving.

Nutrition: Cal: 50, Carbs: 4g Net Carbs: 2.5 g, Fiber: 4.5 g, Fat: 7 g, Protein: 6g, Sugars: 7 g.

4. Cinnamon Almond Flour Bread

Preparation Time: 7 minutes

Cooking Time: 18 min

Serving: 9

Ingredients:

- 2 cups fine whitened almond flour (I utilize Bob's, Red Mill)
- 2 teaspoon coconut flour
- 1/2 teaspoon ocean salt
- teaspoon heating pop
- 1/4 cup Flaxseed supper or chia dinner (ground chia or flaxseed; see notes for how to make your own)
- 5 Eggs and 1 egg white whisked together
    - teaspoon Apple juice vinegar or lemon juice
- teaspoon maple syrup or nectar
- 2–3 teaspoon of explained spread (dissolved) or Coconut oil; separated. Vegetarian margarine likewise works
- 1 teaspoon cinnamon in addition to extra for fixing
- Optional chia seed to sprinkle on the top before preparing

Directions:

1. Preheat stove to 350F. Line an 8×4 bread dish with material paper at the base and oil the sides.
2. In a huge bowl, combine your almond flour, coconut flour, salt, preparing pop, flaxseed feast or chia supper, and 1/2 tablespoon of cinnamon.

3. In another little bowl, whisk together your eggs and egg white. At that point include your maple syrup (or nectar), apple juice vinegar, and dissolved margarine (1.5 to 2 teaspoon).
4. Mix wet fixings into dry. Make certain to expel any bunches that may have happened from the almond flour or coconut flour.
5. Pour hitter into your lubed portion container.
6. Bake at 350° for 30-35 minutes, until a toothpick embedded into the focal point of portion, tells the truth. Mine too around 35 minutes yet I am at elevation.
7. Expel from and broiler.
8. Next, whisk together the other 1 to 2 teaspoon of softened margarine (or oil) and blend it in with 1/2 teaspoon of cinnamon. Brush this over your cinnamon almond flour bread.
9. Cool and serve or store for some other time.

Nutrition: Cal: 200, Carbs: 4g Net Carbs: 1.5 g, Fiber: 4.5 g, Fat: 8 g, Protein: 8g, Sugars: 3 g

5. Keto Banana Almond Bread

Preparation Time: 20 minutes

Cooking Time: 2 hours

Total Time: 2 hours 20 minutes

Servings: 12 slices

Ingredients

- 2 large eggs
- 1/3 cup butter, unsalted
- 1/8 cup almond milk, unsweetened
- 2 medium mashed bananas
- 1/3 cup almond flour
- 0.63 tsp. Stevia extract sugar
- 1 ¼ tsps. Baking powder
- ½ tsp. baking soda
- ½ tsp. salt
- ½ cup chopped nuts

Directions

1. Prepare all the ingredients.
2. Ensure all ingredients are at room temperature. Place the butter, eggs, milk, and mashed bananas in the bread bucket.
3. In a mixing bowl, combine all the dry ingredients and mix well.
4. Pour the dry ingredients in the bread bucket.
5. Set the bread machine in QUICK BREAD then close the lid and let it cook until the machine beeps.

6. Cool the bread before slicing and serving.

Nutrition: Calories: 147 Calories from fat: 90 Total Fat: 10 g Total Carbohydrates: 13 g Net Carbohydrates: 12 g Protein: 2 g

6. Microwave Mug Bread

Preparation Time: 8 minutes

Cooking Time: 15 min

Serving: 10

Ingredients:

- egg
- 1 teaspoon coconut flour
- 1/4 teaspoon preparing powder
- 1 teaspoon spread

Directions:

1. Crack your egg into a microwave-safe ramekin or glass mug and beat it with a fork.
2. Add 1 tbsp. of coconut flour and 1/4 tsp. of preparing powder to the egg, at that point microwave around 1 tbsp. of margarine in a different microwave-safe dish and add it to the blend. At that point blend it well with the fork. The blend ought to be genuinely thick.
3. Pop the dish into the microwave for 90 seconds and be cautious when evacuating it as it will be hot. In the event that the bread doesn't fall directly out when you flip your dish over, pull the sides away with a fork or margarine blade and your bread should come directly out. Cut it down the middle and trim the sides if fundamental.

Nutrition: Cal: 20, Carbs: 4g Net Carbs: 2.5 g, Fiber: 4.5 g, Fat: 6 g, Protein: 7g, Sugars: 3 g.

7. Microwave Flax Bread

Preparation Time: 7 minutes

Cooking Time: 25 min

Serving: 13

Ingredients:

- teaspoon spread
- 1 huge egg
- 4 teaspoon ground flaxseed
- 1/2 teaspoon preparing powder

Directions:

1. Add 1 tbsp. of spread to a microwave-safe ramekin and liquefy it in the microwave (10-20 seconds). Split your egg into the dish with the margarine and beat it with a fork.
2. Add 4 tbsp. of ground flaxseed, 1/2 tsp. of preparing powder, and a spot of salt. At that point blend it well with the fork. The blend ought to be thick, so shake the dish around a piece to even it out.
3. Pop the dish into the microwave for 2 minutes and be cautious when evacuating it as it will be hot. On the off chance that the bread doesn't fall directly out when you flip your dish over, pull the sides away with a fork or margarine blade and your bread should come directly out. Cool it on a rack and cut it down the middle.

Nutrition: Cal: 30, Carbs: 4g Net Carbs: 2.5 g, Fiber: 4.5 g, Fat: 3 g, Protein: 1g, Sugars: 4 g.

8. Keto Milk and Honey Breakfast Loaf

Preparation Time: 2 hours

Cooking Time: 10 minutes

Total Time: 2 hours 10 minutes

Servings: 18 slices

Ingredients

- cup + 1 tbsp. almond milk, unsweetened
- tbsps. honey
- tbsps. melted butter
- 1 ½ tsp. salts
- cups almond flour
- 2 tsps. active dry yeast

Directions

1. Put all ingredients in the bread bucket as listed in the ingredient list.
2. Select the BASIC cycle on your bread machine setting, close the lid then press START.
3. Once the loaf is ready, remove from the machine and place in a cooling rack.
4. Slice and serve with your favorite spread.

Nutrition: Calories: 39 Calories from fat: 27 Total Fat: 3 g Total Carbohydrates: 3 g Net Carbohydrates: 3 g Protein: 1 g

9. Keto Ciabatta Bread

Preparation Time: 120 minutes

Cooking Time: 40 minutes

Total Time: 2 hours 40 minutes

Servings: 6 slices

Ingredients

- cup + 2 tbsps. warm water, divided
- 1 tsp. sugar
- ¼ tsp. dry active yeast
- 1 cup vital wheat gluten
- 1 cup super fine almond flour
- ¼ cup flax seed meal
- ¾ tsp. salt
- 1 ½ tsp. baking powder
- tbsps. extra virgin olive oil
- 1 tbsp. melted butter

Directions

1. In a bowl, combine ½-cup warm water, sugar and yeast. Cover and let it sit for 10 minutes or until frothy.
2. In your bread machine bucket, add the yeast mixture, the remaining ½ cup and 2 tbsps. water and olive oil. Add flour, flax seed, salt, and baking powder. Place the bread bucket back in the bread machine and close the lid.

3. Set the bread machine to DOUGH cycle, close the lid then press the START button. After 10 minutes, stop the bread machine. You will have a very sticky dough.
4. Pour the dough on a floured surface and divide into half before rolling into tube like shape (about 2.5 x 7 inches). Place the cut dough on a greased cookie sheet.
5. Preheat your oven for 2 to 3 minutes at 110 degrees F. Turn the oven off and place the dough inside to rise for 1 hour. After 1 hour, you should have about 3.5 x 8 inches raised dough.
6. Preheat your oven at 350 degrees F to start baking.
7. Brush your raised dough with melted butter, then bake for 15 minutes. Take out of the oven and brush once more with butter before returning inside the oven for another 10 to 15 minutes until the dough's internal temperature reaches 200 degrees F.
8. Once done, let the loaf cool for 1 hour before slicing.
9. Serve with scrambled egg or your favorite jam.

Nutrition: Calories: 286 Calories from fat: 171 Total Fat: 19 g Total Carbohydrates: 9 g Net Carbohydrates: 5 g Protein: 21

10. Protein Keto Bread

Preparation time: 10 minutes

Cooking time: 40 minutes

Servings: 12

Ingredients:

- 1/2 cup unflavored protein powder
- 6 tbsp. almond flour
- 5 pastured eggs, separated
- tbsp. coconut oil
- 1 tsp. baking powder
- 1 tsp. xanthan gum
- 1 pinch Himalayan pink salt
- 1 pinch stevia (optional)

Direction:

1. Start by preheating the oven to 325 degrees F.
2. Grease a ceramic loaf dish with coconut oil and layer it with parchment paper.
3. Add egg whites to a bowl and beat well until it forms peaks.
4. In a separate bowl, mix the dry ingredients together.
5. Mix wet ingredients in another bowl and beat well.
6. Fold in dry mixture and mix well until smooth.
7. Fold in the egg whites and mix evenly.
8. Spread the bread batter in the prepared loaf pan.

9. Bake the bread for 40 minutes or until it's done.
10. Slice into 12 slices and serve.

Nutrition: Calories 165 Total Fat 14 g Saturated Fat 7 g Cholesterol 632 mg Sodium 497 mg Total Carbs 3 g Fiber 3 g Sugar 1 g Protein 5 g

11. Super Seed Bread

Preparation Time: 5 minutes

Cooking Time: 22 min

Serving: 7

Ingredients:

- 2/3 cup entire psyllium husk
- 1/4 cup chia seeds
- 1/4 cup pumpkin seeds
- 1/4 cup hemp or sunflower seeds
- Teaspoon ground sesame seeds or ground flaxseeds 1 teaspoon preparing powder
- 1/4 teaspoon salt
- Teaspoon coconut oil
- 1/4 cups fluid egg
- 1/2 cup unsweetened almond milk

Directions:

1. In a huge blending bowl, include every single dry fixing and blend well. You can make your own ground sesame seeds by mixing them until they're a fine powder.
2. Melt the coconut oil in the microwave (around 30 seconds), add it to the dry blend and mix well. At that point include 1/4 cups fluid egg whites and 1/2 cup unsweetened almond milk. Blend well and let the blend represent 10-15 minutes while you preheat your stove to 325° F.

3. Wet some material paper under warm water and shake it off, at that point press it into a 9" x 5" bread tin. Include your blend and press it into the edges of the tin. You can likewise add some additional seeds to the highest point of the blend here. Trim the abundance material paper and put it in the stove for 70 minutes.
4. Slice the whole portion and let cool on a drying rack. This bread can empty if not cut at the earliest opportunity and left to cool on a rack.

Nutrition: Cal: 70, Carbs: 4g Net Carbs: 2.5 g, Fiber: 4.5 g, Fat: 8 g, Protein: 8g, Sugars: 3 g.

12. Pumpkin Pecan Bread

Preparation Time: 10 minutes

Cooking Time: 3 hours

Servings: 1 loaf, 16 servings

Ingredients

- 1/2 cup milk
- 1/2 cup canned pumpkin
- egg
- tablespoons margarine or butter, cut up
- cups bread flour
- tablespoons packed brown sugar
- 3/4 tsp. salt
- 1/4 tsp. ground nutmeg
- 1/4 tsp. ground ginger
- 1/8 tsp. ground cloves
- 1 tsp. active dry yeast or bread machine yeast
- 3/4 cup coarsely chopped pecans

Direction:

1. Add all ingredients to machine pan.
2. Select basic cycle.

Nutrition: 159 Calories, 6 g total fat (1 g sat. fat), 14 mg, chol, 126 mg sodium, 23 g carb. 1 fiber, 4 g protein

KETO PASTA

13. Chicken Noodle Soup

Preparation Time: 15 minutes

Cooking time: 50 minutes

Servings: 4

Ingredients:

- 3 cups chicken brew (use this recipe or get this) (approx. 720ml).
- 1 chicken bust cut right into small portions (approx. 240g or 0.5 pounds).
- 2 tablespoons avocado oil.
- 1 stalk of celery, sliced (approx. 57g).
- 1 green onion, sliced (approx. 10g).
- 1/4 cup cilantro, finely sliced (approx. 15g).
- 1 zucchini, peeled (approx. 106g).
- Salt to taste.

Directions:

1. Dice the chicken bust.
2. Add the avocado oil right into a pan and sauté the diced chicken in there until cooked.
3. Include chicken broth to the same saucepan as well as simmer.
4. Cut the celery and add it in the pan.
5. Cut the environment-friendly onions as well as include it right into the saucepan.

6. Slice the cilantro as well as put it apart for the moment.
7. To Produce zucchini noodles, I made use of a potato peeler to produce long strands; however, other options consist of using a spiralizer or a food mill with the shredding accessory.
8. Add zucchini noodles as well as cilantro to the pot.
9. Boil for a few more minutes, add salt to taste, as well as offer immediately.

Nutrition: Calories: 310 Sugar: 3 g Fat: 16 g Carbohydrates: 5 g Fiber: 2 g Protein: 34 g.

14. Thai Chicken Pad See Ew

Preparation Time: 15 minutes

Cooking time: 35 minutes

Servings: 4

Ingredients:

- 1 chicken breast (0.5 lb. or 250 g), cut into tiny, thin pieces
- 1/4 cup (0.6 oz. or 17 g) green onion, diced (scallions).
- 1 cup (4 oz. or 115 g) broccoli florets, broken into tiny florets.
- 1 teaspoon fresh grated ginger.
- 1 tablespoon (15 ml) tamari sauce (use coconut aminos for AIP).
- 2 garlic cloves, minced.
- 1 tablespoon cilantro, finely chopped.
- 1 tablespoon (15 ml) coconut oil to cook in.
- 1 cucumber, peeled into long noodles utilizing a potato peeler.
- Salt to taste.

Directions:

1. Break the broccoli up into tiny florets.
2. Cut the chicken breast right into tiny, thin pieces.
3. Grate the ginger, dice the garlic, cut up the environment-friendly onions, as well as cut up the cilantro.
4. Place the coconut oil into a sauté pan.
5. Add in the chicken the green onions and also sauté.
6. Add in the broccoli, ginger, as well as tamari sauce, and then put a lid over the sauté pan, allow let the broccoli chef on

medium heat up until it's tender to your preference (approx. 5-10 mins).

7. Use a potato peeler to develop strands of long cucumber noodles.
8. Split the cucumber noodles between 2 plates.
9. Add to the sauté frying pan the minced garlic, cilantro, as well as salt to preference. Separate and serve in addition to the cucumber noodles.
10. Guidelines.
11. Add one tablespoon of coconut oil right into a huge sauté frying pan and also sauté the chicken breast with onions in it.
12. Add the broccoli, ginger, and tamari sauce. Place a lid over the pan and allow the broccoli chef on medium warmth till it's tender to your liking (approx. 5-10 minutes). Stir on a regular basis.
13. At the same time, peel off the cucumber and later create the cucumber noodles by utilizing a potato peeler to peel the cucumber right into long, vast hairs. Divide the cucumber noodles in between two plates.
14. Contribute to the sauté frying pan, the minced garlic, cilantro, as well as salt to preference. Offer on top of the cucumber noodles.

Nutrition: Calories: 154 Fat: 8 g. Carbohydrates: 1.1 g. Protein: 11 g.

15.Paleo Creamy Tomato Pasta

Preparation Time: 15 minutes

Cooking time: 35 minutes

Servings: 4

Ingredients:

- 2 chicken breasts, cubed
- 2 tablespoons ghee or coconut oil to prepare in
- 1 can diced tomatoes (14 oz or 400g).
- 1/2 cup basil, sliced.
- 1/4 cup coconut milk.
- 6 cloves garlic, minced.
- Salt to taste.
- 1 zucchini, shredded or spiralized (for the pasta) or pasta squash.

Directions:.

1. Sauté the diced chicken in the ghee or coconut oil up until cooked as well as slightly browned.
2. Add the container of diced tomatoes as well as salt to taste. Place on a simmer as well as prepare the liquid down.
3. In the meantime, prepare the pasta. If utilizing zucchinis, shred them in the mixer or.
4. Use a julienne peeler or a spiralizer. If making use of spaghetti squash, slice it in half, remove the seeds, cover gently with some coconut oil and microwave each half for 7 mins.

5. Include the basil, garlic, and also coconut milk to the chicken and cook for a couple of minutes longer.
6. Place half of the pasta right into each dish as well as top with the velvety tomato basil chicken.

Nutrition: Calories: 540 Sugar: 8 g Fat: 27 g Carbohydrates: 1.5 g Fiber: 4 g Protein: 59 g.

16.Goulash with Low Carb Pasta

Preparation Time: 15 minutes

Cooking time: 45 minutes

Servings: 4

Ingredients:

- 1 7 ounce package shirataki ziti noodles
- 1/2 tsp onion powder
- 2 cloves garlic minced
- 1 pound mass sausage
- 14.5 ounce tinned diced tomatoes
- 1/4 cup chopped celery
- 1 packet stevia
- 1 teaspoon salt
- 1 teaspoon chili powder

Directions:

1. Drain shirataki noodles, soak in water for 5 mins, drain once again, then stir fry in a dry pan till noodle feel like they are sticking to the pan.
2. Prepare sausage with onion powder and also garlic until brown.
3. Drain pipes off fat as needed.
4. Include the remaining ingredients.
5. Simmer covered for about 20 minutes, mixing often.

Nutrition: Calories: 540 Sugar: 8 g Fat: 27 g Carbohydrates: 1.5 g Fiber: 4 g Protein: 59 g.

17. Meatball Zoodle Soup

Preparation Time: 15 minutes

Cooking time: 45 minutes

Servings: 4

Ingredients:

- 32 oz. beef supply.
- 1 tool zucchini, Spiraled.
- 2 ribs celery, chopped.
- 1 tiny onion, diced.
- 1 carrot, cut.
- 1 tool tomato, diced.
- 1 1/2 tsp. garlic salt.
- 1 1/2 pound ground beef.
- 1/2 cup Parmesan cheese, shredded.
- 6 cloves garlic, minced.
- 1 large egg.
- 4 tbsp. fresh parsley, sliced.
- 1 1/2 tsp. sea salt.
- 1 1/2 tsp. onion powder.
- 1 tsp. Italian flavoring.
- 1 tsp. dried oregano.
- 1/2 tsp. black pepper.

Directions:

1. Heat slow-moving cooker on the reduced setting.
2. To the sluggish stove, add beef stock, zucchini, celery, onion, carrot, tomato, as well as garlic salt, then cover it.
3. In a big mixing dish, mix hamburger, Parmesan, garlic, egg, parsley, sea salt, onion powder, oregano, Italian seasoning, as well as pepper.
4. Mix till all ingredients are well integrated—kind right into around 30 meatballs.
5. Heat olive oil in a huge skillet over medium-high heat. As soon as the pan is warm, add meatballs and brown on all sides.
6. Add meatballs to slow down cooker, cover, and also cook for 6 hrs.

Nutrition: Calories: 532 Sugar: 5 g Fat: 21 g Carbohydrates: 3.5 g Fiber: 2 g Protein: 25 g.

18.Zucchini Pasta with Bacon Pesto

Preparation Time: 15 minutes

Cooking time: 45 minutes

Servings: 4

Ingredients:

- 10 rashers smoked bacon
- 2 cloves garlic, diced
- 1/4 cup mint leaves, loaded
- 1/2 cup basil leaves, packed
- 3/4 cup flat-leaf parsley, loaded
- 3/4 cup olive oil
- 3 big zucchini
- Fine sea salt to taste

Directions:

1. Preheat the griddle.
2. Lay the bacon rashers on a big baking tray and also broil for 10 to 12 mins until crispy.
3. Transfer to a large plate lined with absorptive kitchen area paper and enable it to cool and solidify.
4. Pour the fat into a small container.
5. When the bacon is crunchy, break rashers into large pieces as well as take into a food processor, together with the remaining pesto components. Blitz up until you have an instead loosened paste with small grain-sized bacon portions for appearance.

6. At the same time, prepare the zucchini noodles. Cut off each zucchini and peel the skin if you desire (I didn't). Making use of a spiralizer or a julienne peeler, make "pasta" from each one, clipping midway to stop them being also long.
7. Heat a tbsp of the reserved bacon fat in a vast sauté frying pan (scheduling any more for another usage), include the zucchini, and cook for around 5 mins on a low-medium warm-up until tender.
8. Put noodles into a bowl-shaped sieve and drain well.
9. Currently, turn off the warm, wipe out the sauté frying pan with cooking area paper as well as return the zucchini to the pan. Add the pesto and also blend well, so the noodles are equally covered.
10. Have a fast taste and add salt if needed, though you may find your bacon makes it salted sufficient.
11. Offer quickly.

Nutrition: Calories: 532 Sugar: 5 g Fat: 21 g Carbohydrates: 3.5 g Fiber: 2 g Protein: 25 g.

19. Sun-Dried Tomato Pesto and Sausage Pasta

Preparation Time: 15 minutes

Cooking time: 50 minutes

Servings: 6

Ingredients:

- 4-5 medium-sized zucchini (or sub pasta of selection).
- 1 lb. Sweet Italian sausage, cases removed.
- 1 onion, diced.
- 1 tbsp. olive oil.
- 1 tablespoon minced garlic.
- For the Pesto.
- 1-8.5 ounce container sun-dried tomatoes in oil.
- 1/4 cup reserved oil from sun-dried tomatoes.
- 1 cup of fresh basil leaves.
- 1/4 cup of fresh parsley.
- 1/2 cup pine nuts.
- 2 tsp. Lemon juice.
- 1-15-oz can diced tomatoes, drained.
- 1/2 tsp oregano.
- 1/2 tsp garlic powder.
- Salt and pepper to taste.
- Garnish.
- Sliced fresh basil and also parsley.

Directions.

1. Spiralize your zucchini and also set aside in a huge pot.
2. In a large frying pan, cook sausage, onion, and also garlic till sausage is browned and well prepared.
3. Drain your sun-dried tomatoes, booking 1/4 cup of oil.
4. In a food mill, incorporate sun-dried tomatoes, basil, parsley, ache nuts, and 1/4 cup reserved oil. Refine up until the herbs, tomatoes, and also nuts have broken up well. Add the remaining to be ingredients and also procedure up until thick as well as somewhat velvety.
5. Add pesto sauce to the frying pan with the sausage and also mix periodically, until warmed.
6. Cook zucchini noodles on tool heat as well as mix sometimes, till softened, concerning 5-7 minutes. Drain pipes excess water.
7. Plate zucchini noodles, top with pesto sausage sauce, and add fresh herbs.

Nutrition: Calories: 347 Sugar: 3 g Fat: 21 g Carbohydrates: 4 g Fiber: 2 g Protein: 54 g.

20. Autoimmune Paleo Spaghetti Squash Chicken Pasta

Preparation Time: 15 minutes

Cooking time: 50 minutes

Servings: 6

Ingredients:

- 1 tool spaghetti squash.
- 1 lb. Boneless skinless chicken breast or upper legs.
- 1 tbsp coconut oil (or various other cooking fat).
- 1 cup basil.
- 1 cup arugula.
- 1/2 cup olive oil.
- one lemon juice.
- 1 clove of garlic, peeled off and also minced.
- Sea salt to taste.

Directions:

1. Preheat the oven to 400 F, and also line two baking sheets with parchment paper.
2. Cook the spaghetti squash as advised.
3. While the pasta squash is baking, add the chicken bust to the various other baking sheets. Add the coconut oil to the hen and period with salt.
4. Cook in the oven for 20-25 mins or up until a thermostat checks out 160 F.

5. When the pasta squash and also chicken are done, scoop the spaghetti squash right into a bowl, top with sliced chicken.
6. For the pesto, add the basil, arugula, olive oil, lemon juice, garlic, and salt to a high-speed blender and also blend till smooth.
7. Top the pasta squash and also chicken with pesto, to enjoy! Store any leftover pesto in the refrigerator for 2-3 days.

Nutrition: Calories: 432 Sugar: 2 g Fat: 32 g Carbohydrates: 3 g Fiber: 3 g Protein: 54 g.

21.AIP Paleo Spaghetti with Meat Sauce

Preparation Time: 15 minutes

Cooking time: 50 minutes

Servings: 6

Ingredients:

- 2 pounds natural turf fed hamburger.
- 1 Tbs. Olive oil.
- 1 1/2 oz cut onions.
- 5-6 cloves of minced fresh garlic or dehydrated minced garlic.
- Sea salt to preference.
- 1 Tbs natural Italian spices.
- 1/2 cup black olives.
- 1 sm container of fresh sliced up mushrooms or 1 can of natural sliced mushrooms.
- 1 bag of natural baby spinach.
- Dietary yeast optional (for cheesy taste).

Directions:

1. Sauté onions & garlic on a medium heat using olive oil, until they become tender & translucent.
2. Add hamburger, sea salt & cook until brown.
3. Add Italian flavoring, olives & mushrooms & cook until mushrooms are done.
4. If you are adding either coconut milk or tomatoes, add them now.
5. Let simmer for about 15-20 minutes.

6. Add spinach.
7. Sprinkle with Nutritional Yeast.
8. Serve over spaghetti squash or glass noodles.

Nutrition: Calories: 432 Sugar: 2 g Fat: 32 g Carbohydrates: 3 g Fiber: 3 g Protein: 54 g.

22. Italian Pasta Salad

Preparation time: 10 minutes

Cooking Time: 2 hours 30 minutes

Serving Size: 12

Ingredients:

- 1/2 teaspoon Italian seasoning
- salt and pepper to taste
- 16 ounces tricolor rotini
- 1/3 cup parmesan cheese (shredded)
- 3 tablespoons parsley (chopped)
- 1/2 red bell pepper (diced)
- 1/3 cup red onion (diced)
- 8 ounces salami (chopped)
- 1/2 green bell pepper (diced)
- 1/2 orange bell pepper (diced)
- 1-pint grape tomatoes (halved)
- 1/2 cup (sliced) black olives
- 1 cup Italian vinaigrette
- 1 cup mozzarella cheese (cubed)

Directions:

1. Make pasta to al dente as per the instructions on the package. In cold water, drain.
2. In a wide container, mix all ingredients. To mix, toss.

3. Before serving, put it in the fridge for at least two hours.

Nutrition: Calories 127 Fat 11, Protein 13 g, Total Carbs 1.3g, Fiber 3g

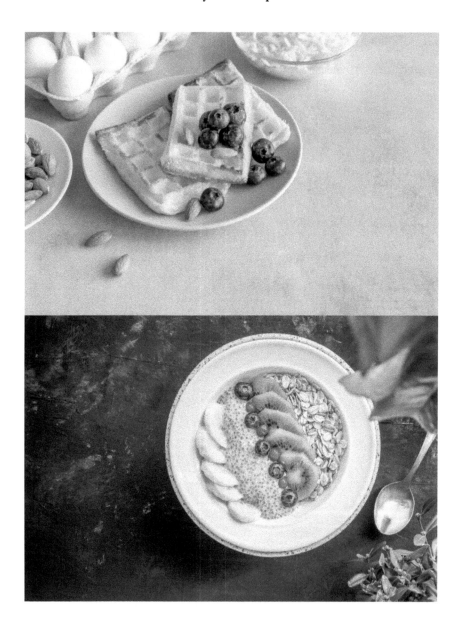

KETO CHAFFLE

23. Buffalo hummus beef chaffles

Preparation time: 15 minutes

Cooking time: 32 minutes

Servings: 4

Ingredients:

- 2 eggs
- cup + ¼ cup finely grated cheddar cheese, divided
- chopped fresh scallions
- Salt and freshly ground black pepper to taste
- chicken breasts, cooked and diced
- ¼ cup buffalo sauce
- tbsp low-carb hummus
- 2 celery stalks, chopped
- ¼ cup crumbled blue cheese for topping

Directions:

1. Preheat the waffle iron.
2. In a medium bowl, mix the eggs, 1 cup of the cheddar cheese, scallions, salt, and black pepper,
3. Open the iron and add a quarter of the mixture. Close and cook until crispy, 7 minutes.
4. Transfer the chaffle to a plate and make 3 more chaffles in the same manner.

5. Preheat the oven to 400 f and line a baking sheet with parchment paper. Set aside.
6. Cut the chaffles into quarters and arrange on the baking sheet.
7. In a medium bowl, mix the chicken with the buffalo sauce, hummus, and celery.
8. Spoon the chicken mixture onto each quarter of chaffles and top with the remaining cheddar cheese.
9. Place the baking sheet in the oven and bake until the cheese melts, 4 minutes.
10. Remove from the oven and top with the blue cheese.
11. Servings afterward.

Nutrition: Calories 552 Fats 28.37g carbs 6.97g net carbs 6.07g protein 59.8g

24. Pulled pork chaffle sandwiches

Preparation time: 20 minutes

Cooking time: 28 minutes

Servings: 4

Ingredients:

- 2 eggs, beaten
- cup finely grated cheddar cheese
- ¼ tsp baking powder
- cups cooked and shredded pork
- tbsp sugar-free bbq sauce
- cups shredded coleslaw mix
- tbsp apple cider vinegar
- ½ tsp salt
- ¼ cup ranch dressing

Directions:

1. Preheat the waffle iron.
2. In a medium bowl, mix the eggs, cheddar cheese, and baking powder.
3. Open the iron and add a quarter of the mixture. Close and cook until crispy, 7 minutes.
4. Transfer the chaffle to a plate and make 3 more chaffles in the same manner.
5. Meanwhile, in another medium bowl, mix the pulled pork with the bbq sauce until well combined. Set aside.

6. Also, mix the coleslaw mix, apple cider vinegar, salt, and ranch dressing in another medium bowl.
7. When the chaffles are ready, on two pieces, divide the pork and then top with the ranch coleslaw. Cover with the remaining chaffles and insert mini skewers to secure the sandwiches.
8. Enjoy afterward.

Nutrition: Calories 374 Fats 23.61g carbs 8.2g net carbs 8.2g protein 28.05g

25. Okonomiyaki chaffles

Preparation time: 20 minutes

Cooking time: 28 minutes

Servings: 4

Ingredients:

- For the chaffles:
- 2 eggs, beaten
- cup finely grated mozzarella cheese
- ½ tsp baking powder
- ¼ cup shredded radishes
- For the sauce:
- tsp coconut aminos
- tbsp sugar-free ketchup
- tbsp sugar-free maple syrup
- tsp worcestershire sauce
- For the topping:
- tbsp mayonnaise
- tbsp chopped fresh scallions
- tbsp bonito flakes
- 1 tsp dried seaweed powder
- 1 tbsp pickled ginger

Directions:

1. For the chaffles:
2. Preheat the waffle iron.

3. In a medium bowl, mix the eggs, mozzarella cheese, baking powder, and radishes.
4. Open the iron and add a quarter of the mixture. Close and cook until crispy, 7 minutes.
5. Transfer the chaffle to a plate and make a 3 more chaffles in the same manner.
6. For the sauce:
7. Combine the coconut aminos, ketchup, maple syrup, and worcestershire sauce in a medium bowl and mix well.
8. For the topping:
9. In another mixing bowl, mix the mayonnaise, scallions, bonito flakes, seaweed powder, and ginger
10. To Servings:
11. Arrange the chaffles on four different plates and swirl the sauce on top. Spread the topping on the chaffles and Servings afterward.

Nutrition: Calories 90 Fats 3.32g carbs 2.97g net carbs 2.17g protein 12.09g

26. Keto reuben chaffles

Preparation time: 15 minutes

Cooking time: 28 minutes

Servings: 4

Ingredients:

- For the chaffles:
- 2 eggs, beaten
- cup finely grated swiss cheese
- tsp caraway seeds
- 1/8 tsp salt
- ½ tsp baking powder
- For the sauce:
- tbsp sugar-free ketchup
- tbsp mayonnaise
- tbsp dill relish
- tsp hot sauce
- For the filling:
- oz pastrami
- swiss cheese slices
- ¼ cup pickled radishes

Directions:

1. For the chaffles:
2. Preheat the waffle iron.
3. In a medium bowl, mix the eggs, swiss cheese, caraway seeds, salt, and baking powder.

4. Open the iron and add a quarter of the mixture. Close and cook until crispy, 7 minutes.
5. Transfer the chaffle to a plate and make 3 more chaffles in the same manner.
6. For the sauce:
7. In another bowl, mix the ketchup, mayonnaise, dill relish, and hot sauce.
8. To assemble:
9. Divide on two chaffles; the sauce, the pastrami, swiss cheese slices, and pickled radishes.
10. Cover with the other chaffles, divide the sandwich in halves and Servings.

Nutrition: Calories 316 Fats 21.78g carbs 6.52g net carbs 5.42g protein 23.56g

27. Pumpkin-cinnamon churro sticks

Preparation time: 10 minutes

Cooking time: 14 minutes

Servings: 2

Ingredients:

- 3 tbsp coconut flour
- ¼ cup pumpkin puree
- egg, beaten
- ½ cup finely grated mozzarella cheese
- tbsp sugar-free maple syrup + more for serving
- tsp baking powder
- tsp vanilla extract
- ½ tsp pumpkin spice seasoning
- 1/8 tsp salt
- 1 tbsp cinnamon powder

Directions:

1. Preheat the waffle iron.
2. Mix all the Ingredients in a medium bowl until well combined.
3. Open the iron and add half of the mixture. Close and cook until golden brown and crispy, 7 minutes.
4. Remove the chaffle onto a plate and make 1 more with the remaining batter.

5. Cut each chaffle into sticks, drizzle the top with more maple syrup and Servings after.

Nutrition: Calories 219 Fats 9.72g carbs 8.64g net carbs 4.34g protein 25.27g

28. Low carb keto broccoli cheese waffles

Preparation time: 5 minutes

Cooking time: 5 minutes

Servings: 2

Ingredients:

- cup broccoli, processed
- cup shredded cheddar cheese
- 1/3 cup grated parmesan cheese
- eggs, beats

Directions

1. spray the Cooking spray on the waffle iron and preheat.
2. Use a powerful blender or food processor to process the broccoli until rice consistency.
3. Mix all Ingredients in a medium bowl.
4. Add 1/3 of the mixture to the waffle iron and cook for 4-5 minutes until golden.

Nutritional: value Calories 160 Total fat 11.8g 18% Cholesterol 121mg 40% Sodium 221.8mg 9% Total carbohydrate 5.1g 2% Dietary fiber 1.7g 7% Sugars 1.2g Protein 10g 20% Vitamin a 133.5µg 9% Vitamin c 7.3mg 12%

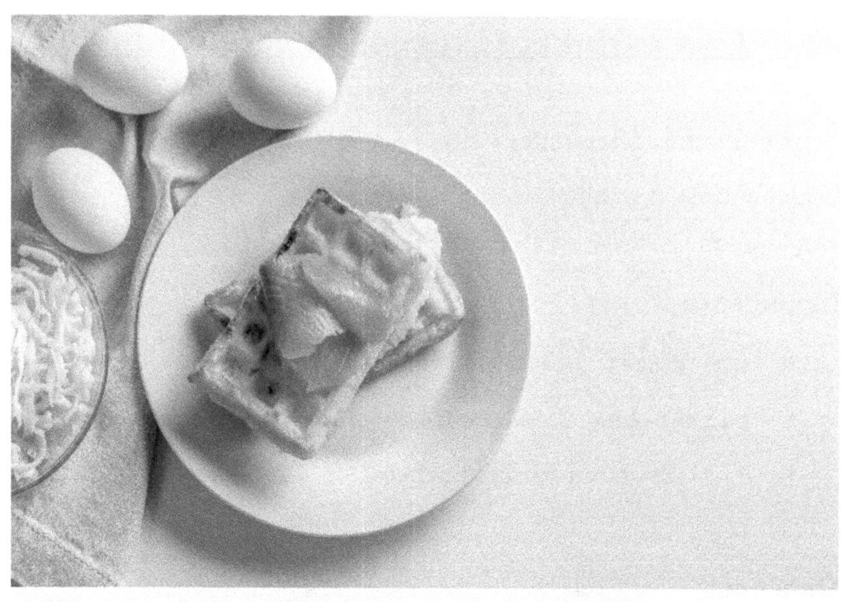

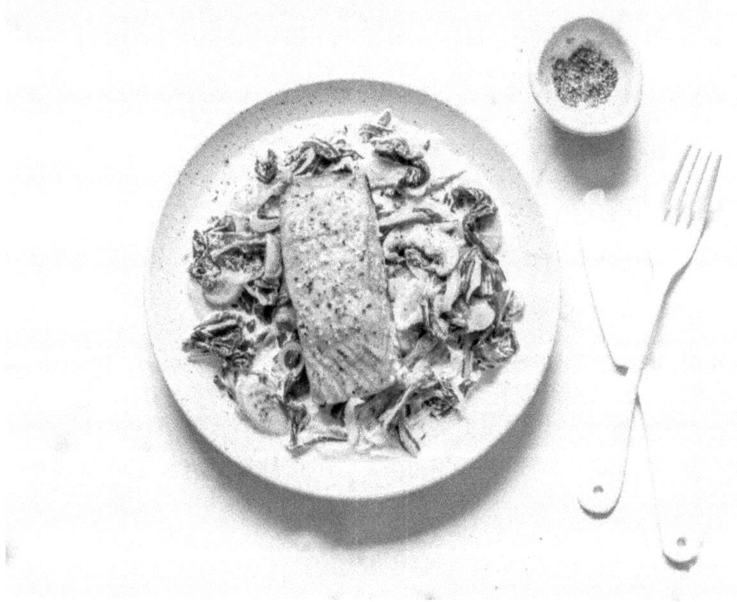

KETO BREAD MACHINE

29. Zucchini Bread

Preparation Time: 1 hour 10 minutes

Cooking Time: 0 minutes

Servings: 16 slices

Ingredients:

- 20 oz. almond flour
- 4 oz. olive oil
- 3 eggs
- 1 tsp. vanilla extract
- 12 oz. erythritol
- 1/8 tbsp. nutmeg
- 1 tsp. cinnamon (ground)
- 1/4 tsp. ginger (ground)
- 8 oz. zucchini (grated)
- 4 oz. walnuts (chopped)
- 1/2 tsp. salt
- 2tsp. of baking powder

Directions:

1. Prepare the oven for baking and heat it to a temperature of 350 degrees Fahrenheit. Whisk the eggs, vanilla extract, and oil in one bowl. Keep them aside.
2. Mix almond flour, salt, nutmeg, ginger, cinnamon, baking powder, and erythritol in a separate bowl.

3. By means of a paper towel or cheesecloth, remove the extra water from zucchini. Then mix the zucchini with the whisked egg mixture.
4. After that, add the mixture of dry items into it. Blend with a hand mixer.
5. Spray some cooking spray on a nine-by-five loaf pan. Use a spoon to put the zucchini mixture into the pan.
6. Put the walnuts on it. Press them by a spatula so that they get embedded in the batter.
7. Bake for 60 to 70 minutes. By then the walnuts should have become slightly brown.

Nutrition: Calories: 200.13 Fat: 18.83 grams Net carbohydrates: 2.6 grams Protein: 5.59 grams

MAINS

30. Cheesy Ham Quiche

Preparation Time: 10 minutes

Cooking Time: 30 minutes

Servings: 6

Ingredients:

- Eggs - 8
- Zucchini - 1 C.,
- Shredded eavy Cream - .50 C.
- Ham - 1 C., Diced
- Mustard - 1 t.
- Salt – Dash

Directions:

1. For this recipe, you can start off by prepping your stove to 375 and getting out a pie plate for your quiche.
2. Next, it is time to prep the zucchini. First, you will want to go ahead and shred it into small pieces.
3. Once this is complete, take a paper towel and gently squeeze out the excess moisture. This will help avoid a soggy quiche.
4. When the step from above is complete, you will want to place the zucchini into your pie plate along with the cooked ham pieces and your cheese.

5. Once these items are in place, you will want to whisk the seasonings, cream, and eggs together before pouring it over the top.
6. Now that your quiche is set, you are going to pop the dish into your stove for about forty minutes.
7. By the end of this time, the egg should be cooked through, and you will be able to insert a knife into the center and have it come out clean.
8. If the quiche is cooked to your liking, take the dish from the oven and allow it to chill slightly before slicing and serving.

Nutrition: Fats: 25g Carbs: 2g Proteins: 20g

31. Feta and Cauliflower Rice Stuffed Bell Peppers

Preparation Time: 10 minutes

Cooking Time: 20 minutes

Servings: 3

Ingredients:

- green Bell Pepper
- red Bell Pepper
- yellow Bell Pepper
- ½ cup Cauliflower rice
- 1 cup Feta cheese
- 1 Onion, sliced
- Tomatoes, chopped
- 1 tbsp black Pepper
- 2-3 Garlic clove, minced
- tbsp Lemon juice
- 3-4 green Olives, chopped
- 3-4 tbsp Olive oil
- Yogurt Sauce:
- 1 clove Garlic, pressed
- 1 cup greek Yogurt
- kosher Salt, to taste
- juice from 1 Lemon

- 1 tbsp fresh Dill

Directions:

1. Grease the Instant Pot with olive oil. Make a cut at the top of the bell peppers near the stem. Place feta cheese, onion, olives, tomatoes, cauliflower rice, salt, black pepper, garlic powder, and lemon juice into a bowl; mix well.
2. Fill up the bell peppers with the feta mixture and insert in the Instant Pot. Set on Manual and cook on High pressure for 20 minutes. When the timer beeps, allow the pressure to release naturally for 5 minutes, then do a quick pressure release.
3. To prepare the yogurt sauce, combine garlic, yogurt, lemon juice, salt, and fresh dill.

Nutrition: Calories 388, Protein 13.5g, Net Carbs 7.9g, Fat 32.4g

32. Beets with Yogurt

Preparation Time: 10 minutes

Cooking Time: 40 minutes

Servings: 3 to 4

Ingredients:

- lb Beets, washed
- Lime, zested and juiced
- cup Plain Full Milk Yogurt
- 1 clove Garlic, minced
- Salt to taste
- 1 tbsp Fresh Dill, chopped
- 1 tbsp Olive oil to drizzle
- Black Pepper to garnish
- 1 cup Water

Directions:

1. Pour the water in the Instant Pot and fit in a steamer basket. Add the beets, seal the lid, secure the pressure valve and select Manual mode on High Pressure mode for 30 minutes.
2. Once ready, do a natural pressure release for 10 minutes, then quickly release the remaining pressure. Remove the beets to a bowl to cool, and then remove the skin. Cut into wedges.
3. Place beets in a dip plate, drizzle the olive oil and lime juice over; set aside. In a bowl, mix garlic, yogurt and lime zest. Pour over the beets and garnish with black pepper, salt, and dill.

Nutrition: Calories 102, Protein 5.7g, Net Carbs 8.2g, Fat 3.8g

SIDES

33. Maple Syrup Bacon

Preparation Time: 5 minutes

Cooking Time: 10 minutes

Servings: 2

Ingredients:

- Maple syrup.
- Thick bacon slices, 11.

Directions:

1. Preheat your pan to 400°F.
2. Place the bacon on the flat surface and brush with the maple syrup.
3. Move to the pan to cook for 10 minutes.
4. Serve and enjoy!

Nutrition: Calories: 91 Carbs: 0g Protein: 8g Fat: 2g

34. Coconut Gratin

Preparation Time: 10 minutes

Cooking Time: 50 minutes

Servings: 8

Ingredients:

- 3 tablespoons olive oil
- 3 garlic cloves, minced
- tablespoon balsamic vinegar
- 1/3 cup coconut cream
- A pinch of salt and black pepper
- tablespoons marjoram, chopped
- ½ cup parmesan, grated
- pounds tomatoes, sliced
- Cooking spray

Directions:

1. Heat up a pan with the olive oil over medium heat, add the garlic, stir and cook for 2 minutes.
2. Add the vinegar, coconut cream, salt, pepper and marjoram, stir and cook for 3 minutes more.
3. Grease baking dish with cooking spray and arrange the tomato slices.

4. Pour the coconut cream mix all over, spread, sprinkle parmesan on top, introduce in the oven and bake at 400 degrees F for 45 minutes.
5. Divide the gratin between plates and serve as a side dish.

Nutrition: Calories: 251 Fat: 3 Fiber: 7 Carbs: 12 Protein: 9

35. Creamy Coleslaw

Preparation Time: 10 minutes

Cooking Time: 2 minutes

Servings: 2

Ingredients:

- 3 ounces green cabbage
- ounce red cabbage
- ounces cucumber
- 6 black olives
- tablespoon scallions
- tablespoons mayonnaise
- ½ tablespoon lemon juice
- tablespoon dill
- 1 tablespoon parsley
- Salt to taste

Directions:

1. Cut the red and green cabbage, olives, scallions, and cucumber into bite-sized pieces and add them to a bowl. Add some salt.
2. Put the lemon juice and mayo in another bowl. Mince the parsley and dill and combine them in.

3. Mix the wet and dry ingredients so you can prepare coleslaw. You can wait for the mixture to marinate a little bit and leave it aside for an hour or simply serve it right away

Nutrition: Calories: 222 Total Carbs: 6g Fiber: 2g Net Carbs: 4g Fat: 21g Protein: 1,5g

VEGETABLES

36. Spinach Salad with Feta Dressing

Preparation time: 5 minutes

Cooking time: 3 minutes

Servings: 2

Ingredients:

- 4 oz of spinach leaves
- 3 tbsp avocado oil
- 3 oz feta cheese, crumbled
- ½ tbsp apple cider vinegar
- 1/8 tsp salt
- 1/8 tsp ground black pepper

Directions:

1. Take a skillet pan, place it over medium heat, add oil and when warmed, add cheese, cook for 1 minute until cheese has slightly melted and then stir in vinegar; remove the pan from heat.
2. Take a bowl, add spinach in it, top with feta cheese mixture and toss until mixed.
3. Serve.

Nutrition: 204.3 Calories; 19.5 g Fats; 5.1 g Protein; 1.7 g Net Carb; 0.8 g Fiber;

37. Salad Sandwiches

Preparation time: 5 minutes

Cooking time: 0 minutes

Servings: 2

Ingredients:

- 2 cabbage leaves
- avocado, pitted
- 1-ounce butter, unsalted
- oz feta cheese, sliced, full-fat

Directions:

1. Divide cabbage leaves into two parts, then smear them with butter and top with cheese.
2. Cut avocado in half, remove the pit, scoop out the flesh and then top it onto each cabbage.
3. Roll the cabbage and then Serve.

Nutrition: 187 Calories; 42.5 g Fats; 5 g Protein; 1.5 g Net Carb; 4 g Fiber;

38. Garlic Butter Zucchini Noodles

Preparation time: 5 minutes

Cooking time: 5 minutes;

Servings: 2

Ingredients:

- 2 medium zucchini
- 2 tsp dried cilantro
- ½ of a lime, juiced
- 2 tbsp butter, unsalted
- 2 tbsp avocado oil
- 2/3 tbsp Sriracha sauce
- 1/3 tsp red chili flakes
- ¼ tsp salt
- ¼ tsp ground black pepper

Directions:

1. Prepare zucchini noodles and for this, trim the ends of zucchini and then spiralize them by using a vegetable peeler or a spiralizer.
2. Take a medium skillet pan, place it over medium heat, add butter and oil and when the butter melts, add 1 tsp cilantro, lime juice, Sriracha sauce, and red pepper flakes, stir until mixed and cook for 1 minute until fragrant.
3. Add zucchini noodles, toss until coated, and then cook for 3 minutes until tender-crisp.

4. Season with salt and black pepper, then distribute zucchini between two plates, top with remaining cilantro and then serve.

Nutrition: 287 Calories; 25.5 g Fats; 2.9 g Protein; 7.6 g Net Carb; 3.9 g Fiber;

SOUPS AND STEWS

39. Potato Cauliflower Leek Soup

Preparation Time: 15 minutes

Cooking Time: 30 minutes

Servings: 6

Ingredients:

- 2 tablespoons olive oil
- 3 leeks, halved lengthwise and chopped
- 4 garlic cloves, minced
- 2 large russet potatoes, peeled and cut into a small dice
- 2 cauliflower heads, cut into small florets (about 5 cups)
- 5 cups Classic Vegetable Broth
- 3 thyme sprigs
- 2 bay leaves
- cup nondairy milk of choice
- Salt
- Black pepper
- tablespoons chopped chives for garnish

Directions:

1. In a large pot, heat the olive oil over medium-high heat. Add the leeks, garlic, and sauté for 3 minutes.
2. Add the potatoes and cauliflower and stir to combine. Add the broth, thyme, and bay leaves and bring to a boil, making

sure all the vegetables are fully submerged in the broth. Then reduce the heat and simmer for 25 minutes, until the cauliflower and potatoes are fork tender. Remove the thyme and bay leaves.

3. Using an immersion blender, purée the soup until creamy. Stir in the nondairy milk. If a thinner soup consistency is desired, add more milk or broth and purée until the desired consistency is reached. Alternatively, add the soup to a high-speed blender in small batches to purée.
4. Season with salt and pepper to taste. Garnish with the chives.

Nutrition: Calories: 250 Fat: 6g Protein: 9g Cholesterol: 0mg Sodium: 230mg Carbohydrates: 43g Fiber: 7g

40. Split Pea Soup

Preparation Time: 20 minutes

Cooking Time: 2 hours

Servings: 6

Ingredients:

- Freezer friendly, gluten-free, vegan, dairy-free
- 2 tablespoons olive oil
- 2 medium onions, chopped
- 2 carrots, peeled and chopped
- 3 celery stalks, chopped
- 2 cups green split peas
- ½ teaspoon dried basil
- teaspoon ground cumin
- ½ teaspoon gram masala
- bay leaves
- 6 cups Classic Vegetable Broth
- cup water
- Salt
- Black pepper

Directions:

1. In a large pot, heat the olive oil over medium-high heat. Add the onions, carrots, and celery. Sauté until the onions are translucent and the vegetables are tender, 5 to 7 minutes.
2. Stir in the split peas, basil, cumin, gram masala, and bay leaves.

3. Add the broth and stir to combine. Bring to a boil, and then reduce to a low simmer. Cover and cook for 1½ hours, stirring every 30 minutes, until the peas are tender.
4. Stir and adjust the consistency by adding ½ cup of water at a time.
5. Remove the bay leaves. Season with salt and pepper to taste.

Nutrition: Calories: 230 Fat: 4.5g Protein: 16g Cholesterol: 0mg Sodium: 240mg Carbohydrates: 45g Fiber: 18g

DRESSING AND SAUCES

41. Pizza Sauce

Preparation Time: 15 minutes

Cooking Time: 45 minutes

Servings: 8

Ingredients:

- 2 tablespoons olive oil
- 2 anchovy fillets
- 2 tablespoons fresh oregano leaves, finely chopped
- 3 garlic cloves, minced
- ½ teaspoon dried oregano, crushed
- ½ teaspoon red pepper flakes, crushed
- (28-ounces) can whole peeled tomatoes, crushed
- ½ teaspoon Erythritol
- Salt, as required
- Pinch of freshly ground black pepper
- Pinch of organic baking powder

Directions:

1. Warm the oil in a medium pan at medium-low heat and cook the anchovy fillets for about 1 minute, stirring occasionally.
2. Stir in the fresh oregano, garlic, dried oregano, and red pepper flakes and sauté for about 2-3 minutes.

3. Add the remaining ingredients except for baking powder and bring to a gentle simmer.
4. Lower the heat, then simmer for about 35-40 minutes, stirring occasionally.
5. Stir in the baking powder and remove from heat.
6. Place on room temperature to cool completely before serving.
7. You can preserve this sauce in the refrigerator by placing it into an airtight container.

Nutrition: Calories: 56 Net Carbs: 3.4g Carbohydrate: 5.1g Fiber: 1.7g Protein: 1.4g Fat: 4g Sugar: 2.7g Sodium: 61mg

DESSERT

42. Strawberry Ice Cream

Preparation time: 2 hours and 5 minutes

Cooking time: 0

Servings: 6

Ingredients:

- cup heavy whipping cream
- 1/3 cup erythritol
- large egg yolks
- ½ tsp vanilla extract
- 1/8 tsp xanthan gum
- tbsp vodka
- cup strawberries, pureed

Directions:

1. Add cream to a pot and place it over low heat and warm it up.
2. Stir in 1/3 cup erythritol and mix well to dissolve.
3. Beat in egg yolks and continue whisking until fluffy.
4. Stir in vanilla extract and mix well until smooth.
5. Lastly, add 1/8 tsp xanthan gum and the vodka.
6. Mix well then transfer the mixture to an ice cream machine and churn as per the machine's instructions.

7. Freeze it for 1 hour then add pureed strawberries.
8. Churn again and freeze for another 1 hour.
9. Serve.

Nutrition: Calories 259 Total Fat 34 g Saturated Fat 10.3 g Cholesterol 112 mg Sodium 92 mg Total Carbs 8.5 g Sugar 2 g Fiber 1.3 g Protein 7.5 g

43. Keto Vanilla Ice Cream

Preparation time: 8 hours and 5 minutes

Cooking time: 0

Servings: 8

Ingredients:

- 2 15-oz cans coconut milk
- 2 cup heavy cream
- ¼ cup Swerve confectioner's sweetener
- tsp pure vanilla extract
- Pinch kosher salt

Directions:

1. Refrigerate coconut milk for 3 hours or overnight and remove the cream from the top while leaving the liquid in the can. Place the cream in a bowl.
2. Beat the coconut cream using a hand mixer until it forms peaks.
3. Stir in vanilla, sweeteners, and whipped cream then beat well until fluffy.
4. Freeze this mixture for 5 hours.
5. Enjoy.

Nutrition: Calories 255 Total Fat 23.4 g Saturated Fat 11.7 g Cholesterol 135 mg Sodium 112 mg Total Carbs 2.5 g Sugar 12.5 g Fiber 1 g Protein 7.9 g

44. Butter Pecan Ice Cream

Preparation time: 5 minutes

Cooking time: 5 minutes

Servings: 3

Ingredients:

- ½ cups unsweetened coconut milk
- ¼ cup heavy whipping cream
- 5 tbsp butter
- ¼ cup crushed pecans
- 25 drops liquid stevia
- ¼ tsp xanthan gum

Directions:

1. Place a pan over medium-low heat and melt butter in it until it turns brown.
2. Mix this butter with chopped pecans, heavy cream, and stevia in a bowl.
3. Stir in coconut milk then xanthan gum and mix well until fluffy.
4. Add this mixture to an ice cream machine and churn as per the machine's instructions.
5. Once done, serve.

Nutrition: Calories 251 Total Fat 24.5 g Saturated Fat 14.7 g Cholesterol 165 mg Sodium 142 mg Total Carbs 4.3 g Sugar 0.5 g Fiber 1 g Protein 5.9 g

45. Almond Meal Cupcakes

Preparation time: 15 minutes

Cooking time: 15 minutes

Servings: 12

Ingredients:

- ½ cup almond meal
- ¼ cup butter, melted
- 2 (8-ounce / 227-g) packages cream cheese, softened
- 2 eggs
- ¾ teaspoon liquid stevia
- teaspoon vanilla extract
- Special equipment:
- A 12-cup muffin pan

Directions:

1. Preheat your oven to 350°F (180°C). Line a muffin pan with 12 paper liners.
2. Thoroughly mix the almond meal with butter in a bowl, then spoon this mixture into the bottoms of each paper liner and press it into a thin crust.
3. Make the cupcakes: Whisk the cream cheese with liquid stevia, eggs, and vanilla extract in a medium bowl. Beat with an electric beater until the mixture is fluffy, creamy and smooth. Spoon this filling over the crust layer in the muffin pan.
4. Bake in the preheated oven until the cream cheese mixture is cooked from the center, for 15 to 17 minutes.

5. Leave the cupcakes to cool at room temperature. Serve immediately or refrigerate to chill for 8 hours, preferably overnight.

Nutrition: calories: 199 fat: 19.1g total carbs: 2.6g fiber: 0.5g protein: 4.7g

46. Almond Cinnamon Cookies

Preparation time: 10 minutes

Cooking time: 15 minutes

Servings: 12

Ingredients:

- 2 cups blanched almond flour
- ½ cup butter, softened
- egg
- ½ cup Swerve
- teaspoon sugar-free vanilla extract
- teaspoon ground cinnamon

Directions:

1. Preheat your oven to 350°F (180°C). Layer a baking sheet with parchment paper.
2. Whisk the almond flour with butter, vanilla extract, Swerve, egg, and cinnamon in a bowl. Mix well until these ingredients form a smooth dough.
3. Make the cookies: Divide the dough and roll it into 1-inch balls on a lightly floured surface. Arrange these balls on the prepared baking sheet and press each ball lightly with a fork to make a criss-cross pattern.
4. Bake these cinnamon cookies in the preheated oven for 12 to 15 minutes, or until their edges turn golden.

5. Allow the cinnamon cookies to cool on the baking sheet for 5 minutes, then transfer them to a wire rack to cool completely before serving.

Nutrition: calories: 92 fat: 7.4g total carbs: 3.0g fiber: 0.1g protein: 3.4g

47. Egg Avocado Cups

Preparation time: 10 minutes

Cooking time: 20 minutes

Servings: 2

Ingredients:

- avocado, halved and pitted
- eggs
- ¼ cup Cheddar cheese, shredded
- Salt and ground black pepper to taste
- tablespoon fresh parsley, chopped

Directions:

1. Preheat your oven to 425°F (220°C).
2. Using a large spoon to scoop the avocado flesh out of the skin on a flat work surface.
3. Place the avocado halves on a greased baking sheet, then crack an egg into each of the halves.
4. Bake in the preheated oven for 15 to 20 minutes until the eggs are completely set.
5. When ready to serve, top with the Cheddar cheese. Season the cups lightly with salt and black pepper.
6. Sprinkle the fresh parsley on top for garnish to serve.

Nutrition: calories: 342 fat: 30.0g total carbs: 9.9g fiber: 6.8g protein: 15.0g

48. Cream Cheese Chocolate Mousse

Preparation time: 10 minutes

Cooking time: 0

Servings: 2

Ingredients:

- 3 ounces (85 g) cream cheese, softened
- ½ cup heavy cream
- teaspoon vanilla extract
- ¼ cup Swerve
- tablespoons cocoa powder
- pinch salt

Directions:

1. Beat the cream cheese in a large mixing bowl with an electric beater until it makes fluffy mixture.
2. Switch the beater to low speed, and add the vanilla extract, heavy cream, salt, Swerve, and cocoa powder to beat for 2 minutes until it is completely smooth.
3. Chill in the refrigerator until ready to serve.

Nutrition: calories: 270 fat: 26.4g total carbs: 6.0g fiber: 2.0g protein: 4.2g

49. Keto Cream Cheese Frosted Carrot Mug Cake

Preparation Time: 10 minutes

Cooking Time: 2 minutes

Servings: 2

Ingredients:

- Cake:
- 2 tablespoons almond flour
- tablespoon erythritol
- tablespoon psyllium husk
- tablespoon butter (melted)
- 1 piece large egg (beaten lightly)
- 1 teaspoon cinnamon
- 1/2 teaspoon vanilla extract
- 1/2 teaspoon baking powder
- 1/2 piece small carrot (grated finely)
- 1/4 teaspoon ginger (ground)
- pinch of salt
- Frosting:
- 1 tablespoon whipping cream
- 1/4 cup cream cheese (room temperature)
- 1/2 teaspoon vanilla extract
- 1/2 tablespoon erythritol

Directions:

1. In a food processor, put in all the ingredients for the cake. Blend to combine everything.
2. Pour the blended mixture from the food processor into a microwave-safe mug.
3. Microwave it for 90 seconds on high setting.
4. Remove the cake from the mug. Set it aside to cool down.
5. Cut the cake into two layers. Set aside.
6. In a mixing bowl, put in the cream cheese, vanilla extract, and erythritol. Whip them up using an electric hand mixer. Continue whipping until the texture of the mixture becomes soft and creamy.
7. Put in the whipping cream into the cream cheese mixture. Mix thoroughly for 5 minutes.
8. Get the bottom layer of the cake. Scoop a heaping tablespoon of the cream cheese frosting. Spread the frosting on top of the bottom layer of the cake.
9. Get the top layer of the cake. Gently put it on top of the frosted bottom layer of the cake.
10. Spread the rest of the cream cheese frosting on top of the cake and on the sides.
11. You can chill the cake before serving, or you can serve it right away. Cut the cake in half and enjoy.

Nutrition: Calories: 229 Carbs: 20 g Fats: 17.3 g Proteins: 6 g Fiber: 15.9 g

50. Keto Avocado Brownies

Preparation Time: 10 minutes

Cooking Time: 30 minutes

Servings: 12

Ingredients:

- 2 pieces large avocadoes (ripe)
- 100 grams Lily's chocolate chips (melted)
- 4 tablespoons cocoa powder
- 3 tablespoons refined coconut oil
- 1/2 teaspoon vanilla
- 2 pieces eggs
- Dry Ingredients:
- 90 grams almond flour (blanched)
- 1/4 cup erythritol
- teaspoon baking powder
- teaspoon stevia powder
- 1/4 teaspoon baking soda
- 1/4 teaspoon salt

Directions:

1. Preheat your oven to 350 degrees Fahrenheit.
2. In a mixing bowl, put in all the ingredients listed under dry ingredients. Whisk to combine well. Set aside.

3. Cut the avocadoes in half. Scoop out the flesh. Weigh the avocadoes. You will need a total of 250 grams of avocadoes for this recipe.
4. Put the avocadoes in a food processor. Process the avocadoes until the texture becomes smooth.
5. Put in the rest of the ingredients into the food processor one at a time. Process for a few seconds after each ingredient is added into the avocado mixture.
6. Put in the flour mixture into the food processor. Process until everything is well combined.
7. Line a baking dish (12" x 8") with parchment paper. Transfer the avocado batter into the baking dish. Spread the batter evenly on the surface of the baking dish.
8. Bake the batter for 30 minutes. Do the toothpick test to know if the brownie is done. The top surface of the brownie should be soft to the touch.
9. Take the brownie out from the oven. Set it aside to cool down. Cut the brownie into 12 square pieces.

Nutrition: Calories: 155 Carbs: 9.78 g Fats: 14.05 g Proteins: 4.02 g Fiber: 6.98 g

CONCLUSION

Keto can be a great option for people looking to shed extra weight that is stored in their bodies as fat. Ketosis is the process of the body using fats instead of glucose for energy. The liver can take fats and break them down into ketones, which can be used by both the body and the brain as a fuel source. To get the body away from using sugars, however, a person has to severely limit the amount and type of carbs they consume so the body can burn through its glucose stores and start working on the fat stores. This is why it can be so important to stay diligent on the diet once started; otherwise, a person might not see their desired results.

For people who are ready to dedicate themselves 100% to the keto diet, there are various forms of it that can match any person's lifestyle and goals. The standard keto option is best for people trying the diet for the first time because it can be the quickest way to get into ketosis and reap the immediate benefits. There are also cyclical and targeted keto for people who might not be willing to follow the strict diet every day. These options give people an opportunity to consume carbs on certain days based on their own personal plans.

There are many benefits to starting the keto diet beyond just losing weight. Keto can also help people improve their heart health by reducing bad fats and forcing the body to work through fats it has stored, possibly in dangerous places like arteries. It can also help people with certain types of epilepsy reduce seizures by switching the brain onto ketone power. Keto can also help women with PCOS regain their health by promoting weight loss and helping to balance their hormones, which can be a cause of the condition. It can even help clear up acne in some people by reducing blood sugar, which can improve skin conditions.

It is not difficult to switch to and stick to a Keto diet. What is actually difficult is adhering to strict rules and guidelines. As long as you maintain the Fats : Protein : Carbs ratio, you'll lose weight fast. It's a no-brainer. And quite unbecoming that many have deviated from this core principle of the Keto diet. The simple formula is to increase the fat and protein content in your meals and snacks while reducing your carb intake. You must restrict your carb intake to reach and remain in Ketosis. Different people achieve Ketosis with varying amounts of carb intake. Generally, it is easy to reach and stay in Ketosis when you decrease your carb intake to not more than 20grams.

Keeping keto long term can seem difficult for beginners who are just getting used to the mechanics of the diet, but it is not so difficult once they are acclimated to the keto lifestyle. Planning out meals and snacks can help people keep up keto longer because it takes some of the work and thinking out of dieting. A person can simply grab what they need and go. And if the standard keto doesn't work for someone long term, they can refer to the other keto styles to find one that will work for them beyond the initial diet.

Lightning Source UK Ltd.
Milton Keynes UK
UKHW022013080321
380016UK00005B/928